I0136515

Healthy Me

A Simple Guide to Begin Caring for My Whole Self

This journal belongs to:

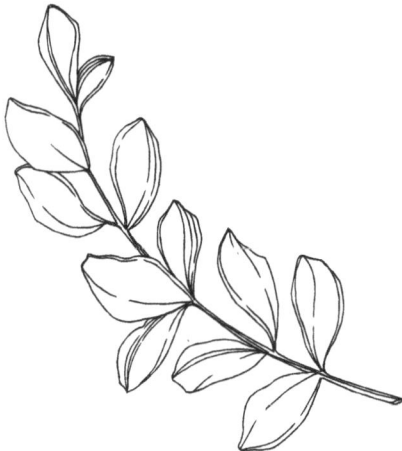

_____

_____

Copyright © 2024 by Rosy Crumpton

All rights reserved. This book may not be reproduced or stored in whole or in part by any means without the written permission of the author except for brief quotations for the purpose of review.

ISBN: 978-1-960146-91-5 (hard cover)
       978-1-960146-92-2 (soft cover)

Edited by: Brody Luna and Amy Ashby

Published by Warren Publishing
Charlotte, NC
www.warrenpublishing.net
Printed in the United States

Warren
publishing

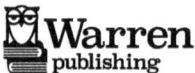

A note from the author

At my deepest core, I identify as a giver.

In my personal life and professional life, I'm a caregiver and really good at it too (not a brag). I sometimes give to my own detriment. Are you a giver too?

Choosing other people's needs before my own is a struggle for me. It's taken a lot of personal internal work to learn why giving is such a big part of who I am. I don't dislike that I'm a giver. I appreciate my life experiences and my innate personality traits that make up who I am. At the same time, I recognize and work on how to be the best healthy version of myself, which includes giving some of that care back to me.

I've learned that a big part of why and how I choose to be a giver is because it's how I wish someone would've taken care of me. This giving system I found myself in was unrealistic, unsustainable, and unfair. While constant giving is personally fulfilling, it can also build resentment, which is terribly unhealthy.

Through personal and professional dedication in wellness, I've learned that meeting my needs is my responsibility and an unfair expectation I shouldn't place on anyone. No one can take care of me like me.

I can now honor the qualities I happen to love about myself and what I value most in my precious, wild life. Focusing on my health—physical, mental, spiritual— is not a selfish endeavor either. It's recognizing I'm part of the beautiful world I've built for myself and that my needs matter too. In my experience, you don't arrive at healed and healthy in a perfect little balanced system either. It's ongoing work.

It is my hope that this journal serves as a useful tool and inspires you to remember to choose yourself and your needs in your beautiful, ever-changing life. Think of it as a free-flowing journal and use it how it best meets your needs. Competing priorities is part of our day-to-day. May this simple guide serve as a reminder that you're a priority and can find your way back to you, your whole healthy self, and your needs. And should you wish my support throughout any of it, contact me and mention this journal.

May it serve you well.

With love,
Rosy Crumpton

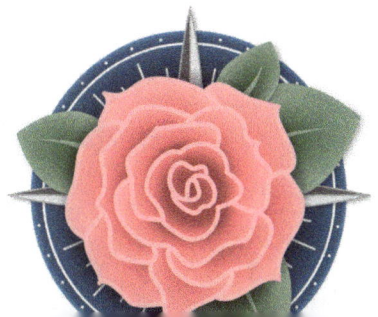

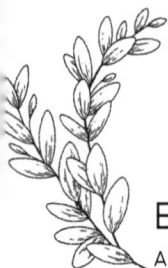

First Things First

Everyone's version of healthy looks different.

Answer the questions below to the best of your ability. Use sentences, words, images, etc. It's your journal and your vision of health. There are no wrong answers.

What does being healthy and well mean to me?

What would life look like if I were living my ideal health?

"Health is a state of complete physical, mental and social well-being and not merely the absence of disease or infirmity."
—World Health Organization

Need another page?

My ideal health continued:

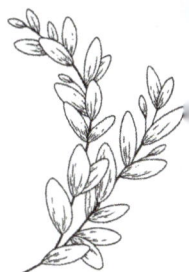

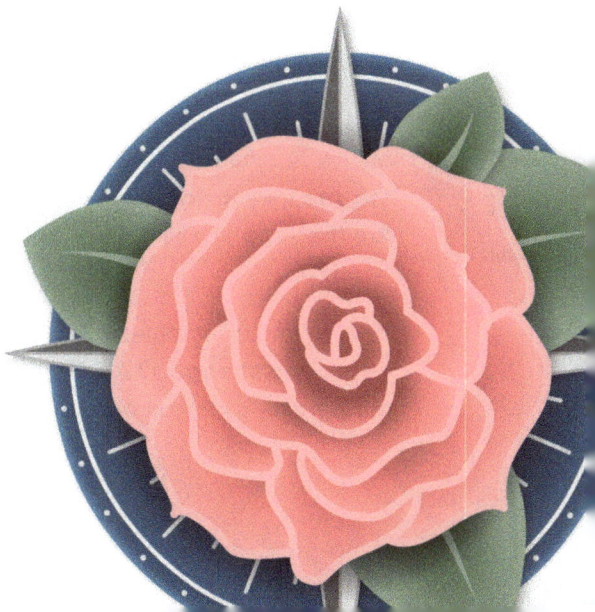

We are whole beings.

When I think about my ideal health, am I considering all aspects of my life that can affect my well-being?

Here are some dimensions of health that impact our wellness.

- **NUTRITION:** What we eat and how we eat. Is it fueling? **Am I honoring my body, food preferences, and needs? Is what I eat boosting my body's natural healing potential?**

- **MOVEMENT:** How we move (exercise). **Is the physical activity I'm engaging in enjoyable and sustainable movement?**

- **REST:** The time we spend to relax and restore energies. **Do I get enough restorative relaxation time? What can I do to maximize my rest?**

- **MENTAL/EMOTIONAL:** How we adapt to our everyday life. **Do I practice healthy tactics to manage day-to-day stressors?**

- **SOCIAL LIFE & RELATIONSHIPS:** Who we spend time with—romantic and non-romantic relationships—and influence. **Are these healthy interactions and experiences that enrich my life?**

- **SPIRITUALITY:** Being connected to something greater, not necessarily affiliated with a religious organization. **Do I have purpose and meaning in something larger than myself?**

- **PHYSICAL ENVIRONMENT:** The physical spaces we operate in from our bedroom to our homes, our neighborhood, our office space, etc. **Are they toxic? Are they safe? Are they organized and clean? Are they operational? Consider noise, safety, clutter, etc.**

- **PERSONAL AND PROFESSIONAL DEVELOPMENT:** What we do is fulfilling and contributes to our stability. **Does it align with our values and strengths? Am I contributing to my community? Am I realizing my personal potential?**

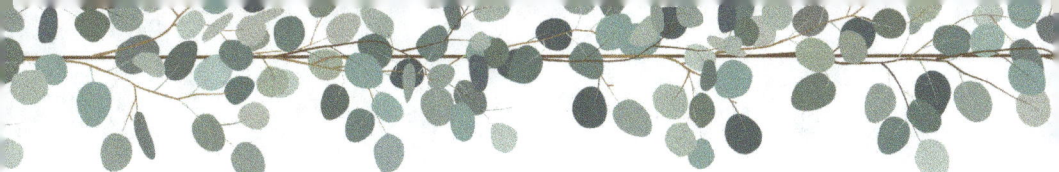

What do I already do To care for myself in These areas?

Nutrition

Movement

Rest

Mental/Emotional

Date: _____

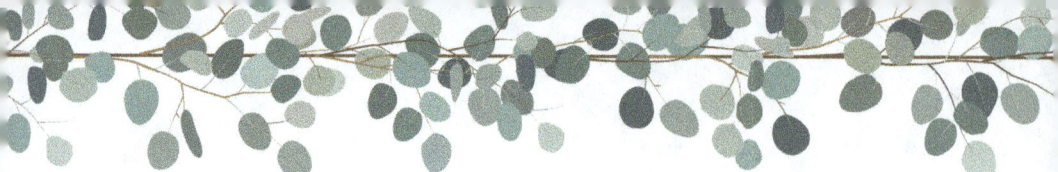

What do I already do to care for myself in These areas?

Social Life & Relationships	Spirituality

Physical Environment	Personal & Professional Development

Date: _____

All my lifestyle components that impact my health and well-being

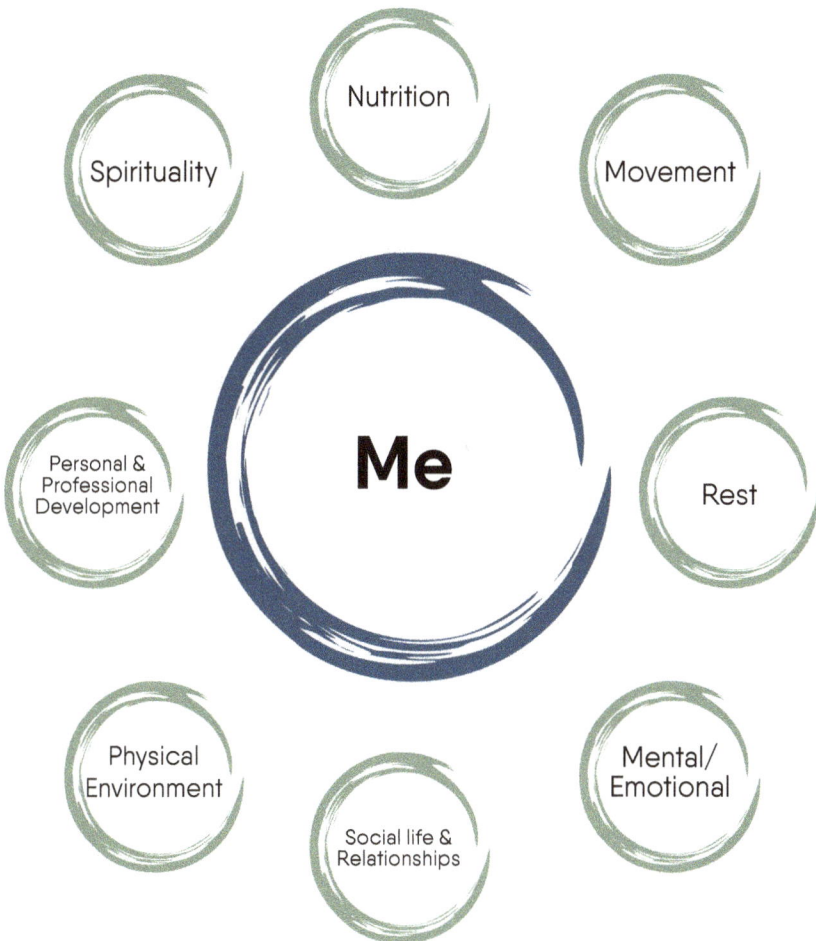

Spirituality

Nutrition

Movement

Personal & Professional Development

Me

Rest

Physical Environment

Social life & Relationships

Mental/ Emotional

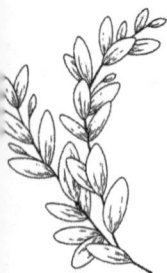

Is there anything not covered under the listed categories?

If so, list on this page and include how I already care for myself in these areas.

Date: _____

What I like about how I currently take care of my needs:

_____

_____

_____

_____

_____

_____

_____

_____

_____

_____

_____

_____

_____

_____

_____

_____

_____

Date: _____

Use this page to document any insight I may have gained from listing how I currently care for my needs.

_____

_____

_____

_____

_____

_____

_____

_____

_____

_____

_____

_____

_____

_____

_____

_____

_____

_____

Date: _____

Date: _____

We are whole beings.

Now that I've thought about how I may already be caring for myself in these areas, is there an area that stands out that I may want to focus a little more on in order to support my well-being?

What area(s) might that be?

Why?

If I were to begin to place more focus on this area, how would I go about it?

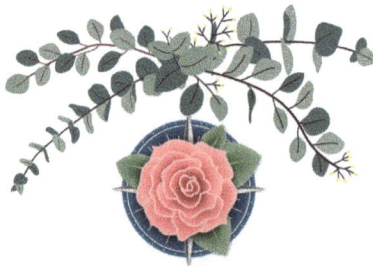

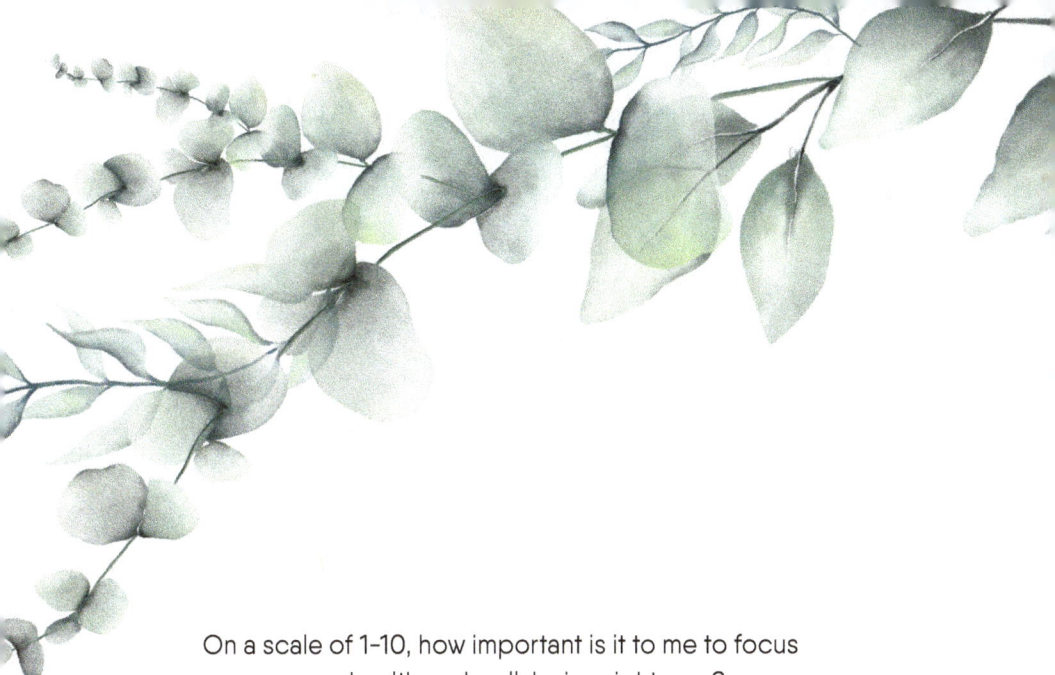

On a scale of 1–10, how important is it to me to focus
on my health and well-being right now?
1 being not important to 10 being most important
(Circle the number that best corresponds).

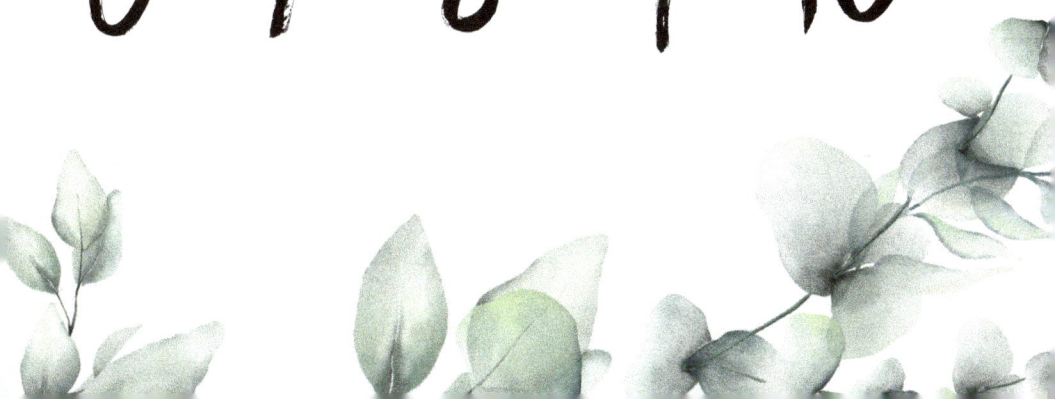

1 2 3 4 5
6 7 8 9 10

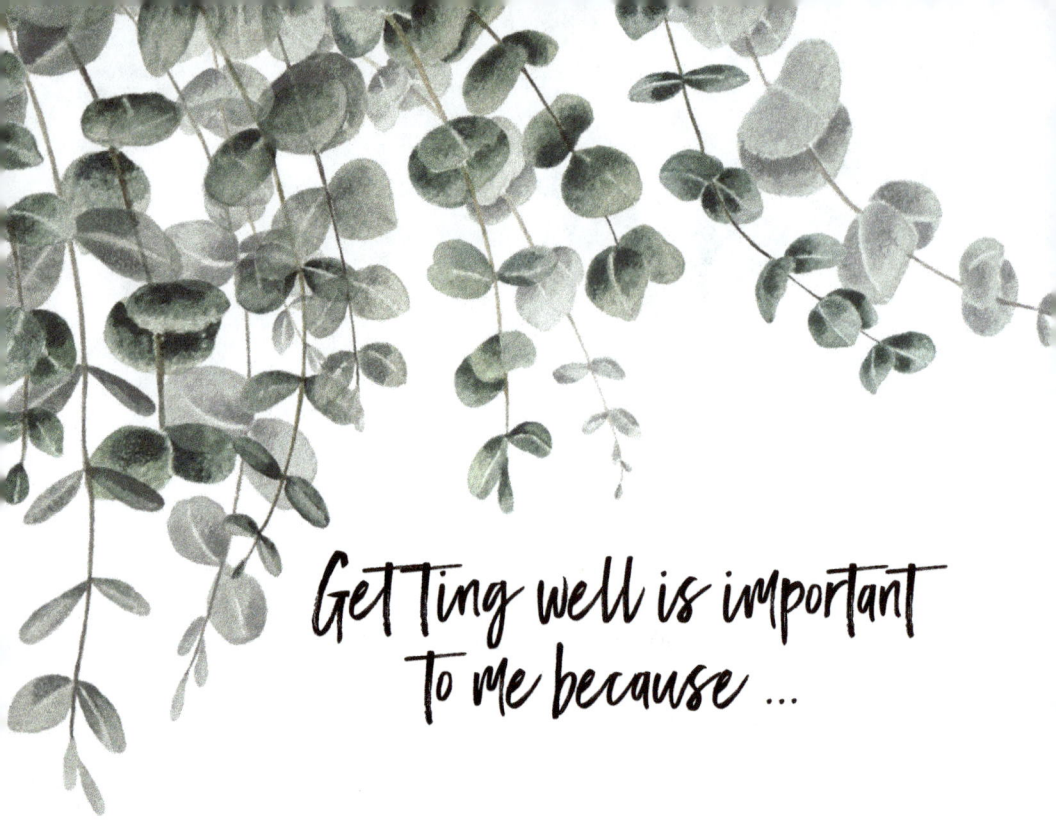

Getting well is important to me because ...

O _____
O _____
O _____
O _____
O _____
O _____
O _____
O _____
O _____
O _____

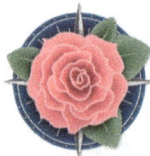

Getting well is important to me because ...

○ _____
○ _____
○ _____
○ _____
○ _____
○ _____
○ _____
○ _____
○ _____
○ _____

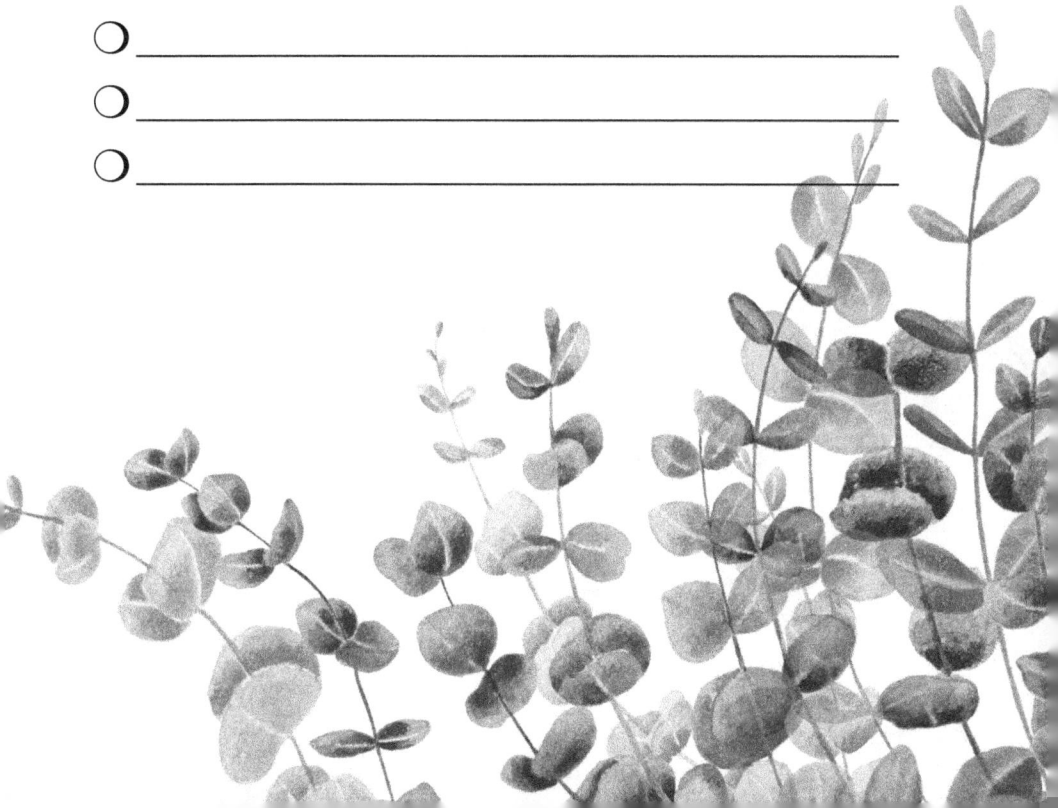

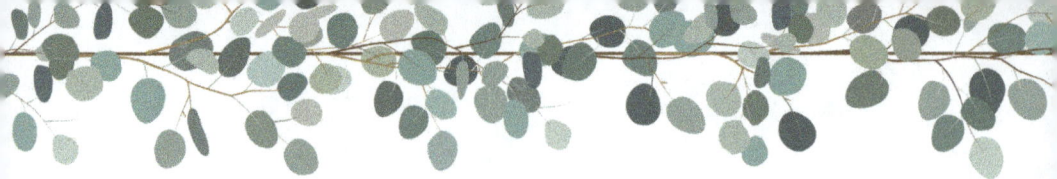

Recognizing and concentrating on our strengths provides insight and supports forward momentum.

- Use the next page to list as many of your strengths as you can think of.

- Think about the unique qualities that make you who you are.

- If needed, ask people around you to tell you what they think your strengths are.

- Take a personality test.

- Write down the qualities you agree and identify are your strengths.

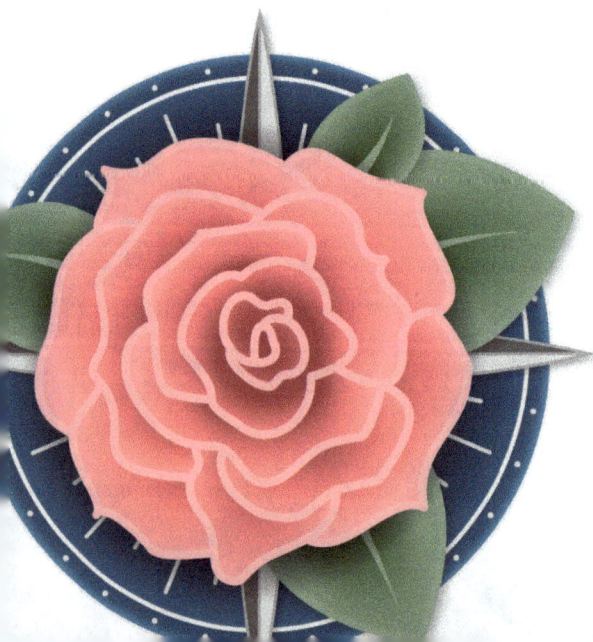

My Strengths

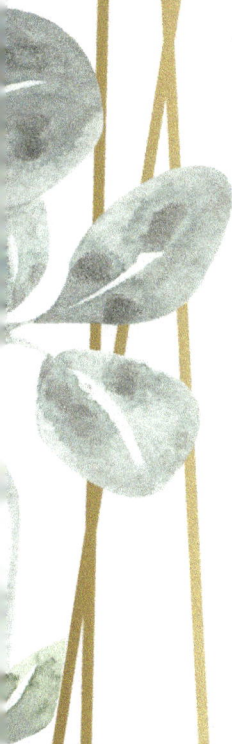

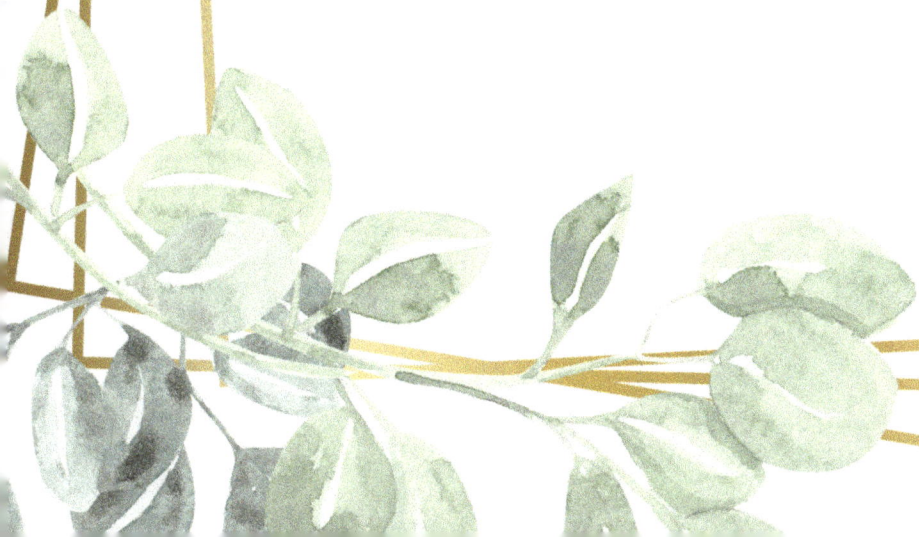

I am:

My Strengths

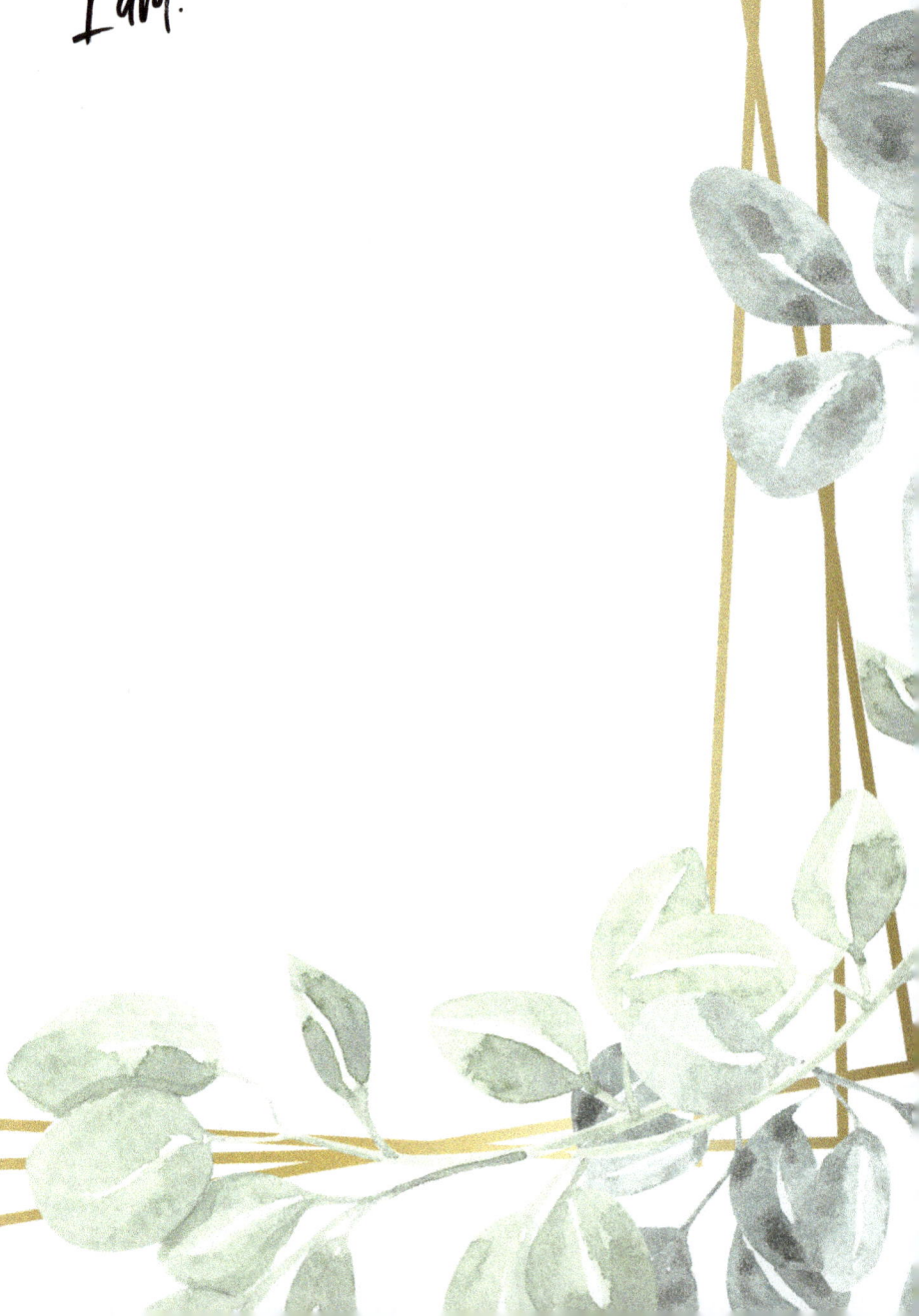

I am:

How will I remember my strengths?

_____

_____

_____

_____

_____

_____

_____

_____

_____

_____

_____

_____

_____

_____

_____

_____

_____

Date: _____

Barriers

What are some of the challenges I experience in terms of my wellness? What gets in the way of me caring more for myself?

If I were to address the barrier(s) above, how might I begin to go about it?

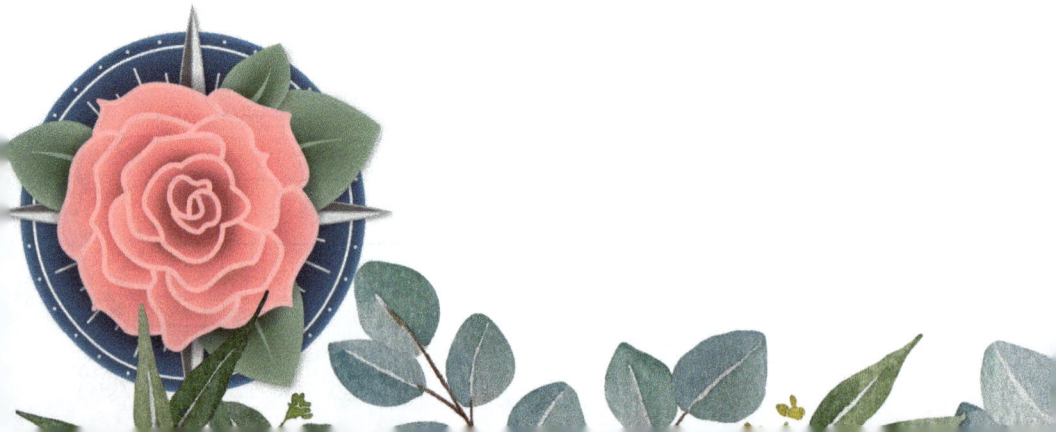

Need another page?

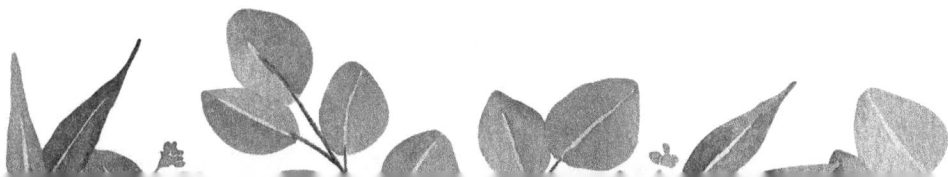

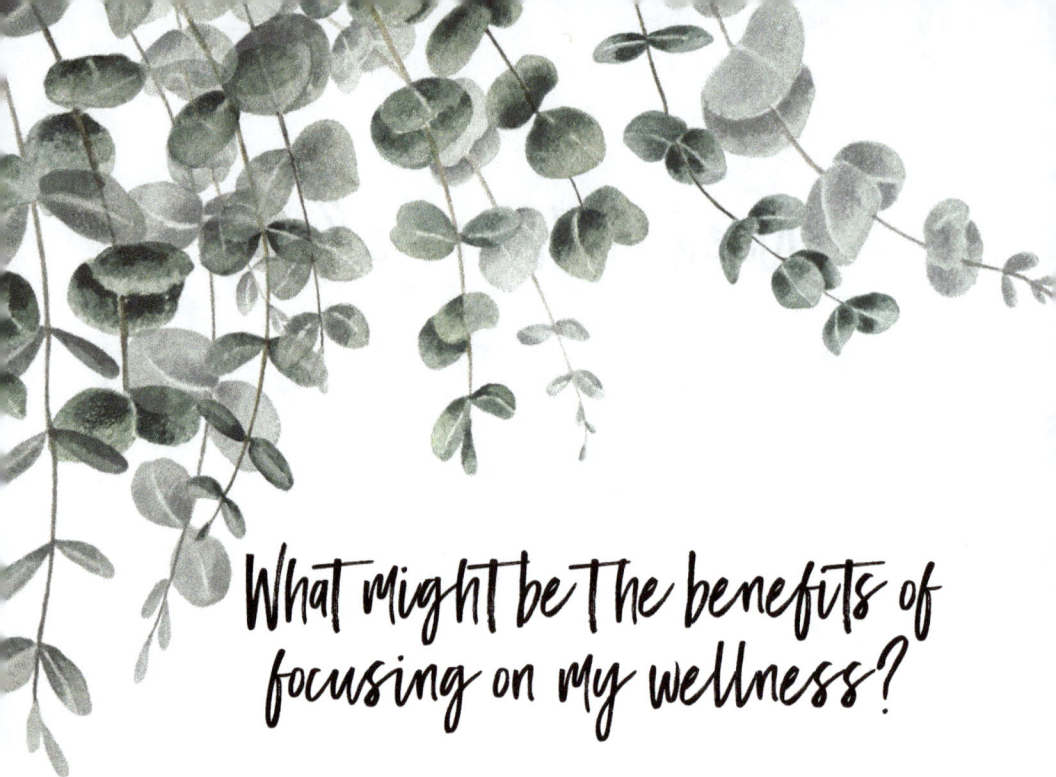

What might be the benefits of focusing on my wellness?

○ _____
○ _____
○ _____
○ _____
○ _____
○ _____
○ _____
○ _____
○ _____
○ _____

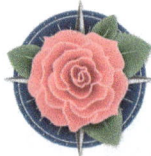

The mind-body connection

When we support our bodies,
we support our minds.

When we support our minds,
we support our bodies.

*Your thoughts lead to your attitudes,
which lead your emotions and can influence your behaviors.
Your behavior leads to habits that affect your physical
and emotional health and well-being as well as your longevity.*

What positive Thoughts can I Turn to when I need To?

Positive affirmations, practicing gratitude, and envisioning your accomplished reality are three powerful tools that might be helpful.

- **POSITIVE AFFIRMATIONS:** A positive and true statement I believe about myself that makes me feel good when I recite it.
  Examples: I am *strong*. I am *smart*. I am *loved*.

- **GRATITUDE PRACTICE:** Taking the time to think about something(s) I am grateful for.
  Challenge: Try to think of something unique about each day and practice as often as needed. Be specific.
  Example: I am grateful for having lunch with my friend Diane today. She really helped energize me.

- **ENVISIONING:** Challenging self to daydream about what could go right and having arrived at the desired outcome.
  Example: Close your eyes and think about what it would feel like to be at the finish line of the anticipated half marathon race.

Positive affirmation ideas

I am focused and disciplined.

I am brave.

I am strong.

I choose my thoughts.

I know my worth.

I am capable.

I am powerful.

I am loved.

I am proud of who I am.

I am true to myself.

I am worthy.

I trust myself.

I am valuable.

I choose to be positive.

I am a magnet for good things.

I am smart.

I am grateful for all that I have.

I am courageous.

I deserve the good that comes into my life.

The positive affirmation that resonates most with me right now is:

_____

_____

_____

_____

_____

Gratitude

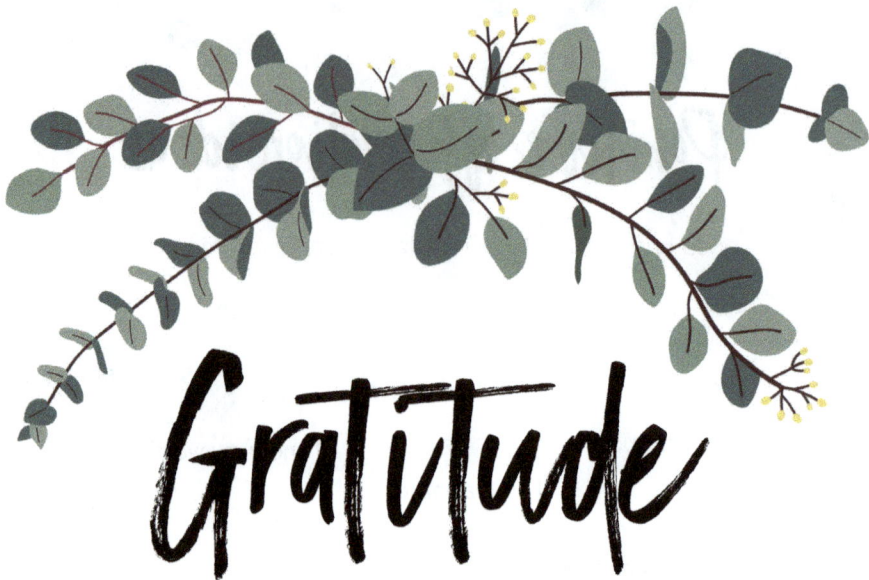

Use this section of your journal for your gratitude practice.

Challenge yourself to practice regularly.

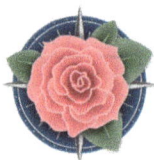

I am grateful for:

Date: _____

_____

_____

_____

_____

_____

_____

_____

Date: _____

_____

_____

_____

_____

_____

_____

_____

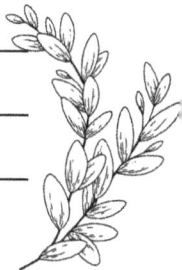

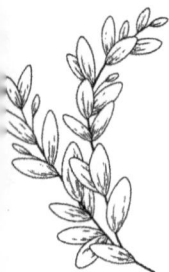

I am grateful for:

Date: _____

_____

_____

_____

_____

_____

_____

_____

_____

Date: _____

_____

_____

_____

_____

_____

_____

_____

I am grateful for:

Date: _____

_____

_____

_____

_____

_____

_____

_____

_____

Date: _____

_____

_____

_____

_____

_____

_____

_____

_____

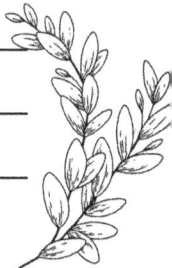

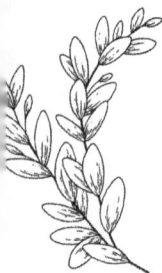

I am grateful for:

Date: _____

_____

_____

_____

_____

_____

_____

_____

Date: _____

_____

_____

_____

_____

_____

_____

_____

I am grateful for:

Date: _____

_____

_____

_____

_____

_____

_____

_____

Date: _____

_____

_____

_____

_____

_____

_____

_____

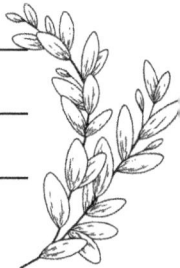

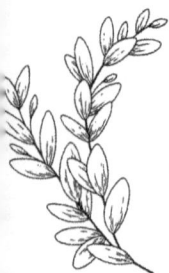

I am grateful for:

Date: _____

_____

_____

_____

_____

_____

_____

_____

Date: _____

_____

_____

_____

_____

_____

_____

_____

I am grateful for:

Date: _____

_____

_____

_____

_____

_____

_____

_____

_____

Date: _____

_____

_____

_____

_____

_____

_____

_____

_____

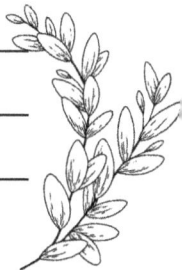

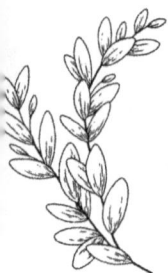

I am grateful for:

Date: _____

_____

_____

_____

_____

_____

_____

_____

Date: _____

_____

_____

_____

_____

_____

_____

_____

I am grateful for:

Date: _____

_____

_____

_____

_____

_____

_____

_____

Date: _____

_____

_____

_____

_____

_____

_____

_____

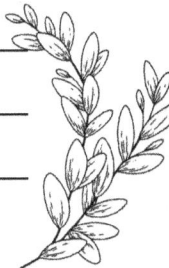

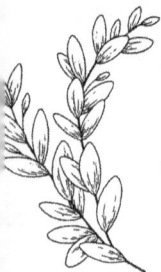

I am grateful for:

Date: _____

_____

_____

_____

_____

_____

_____

_____

_____

Date: _____

_____

_____

_____

_____

_____

_____

_____

_____

I am grateful for:

Date: _____

_____

_____

_____

_____

_____

_____

_____

Date: _____

_____

_____

_____

_____

_____

_____

_____

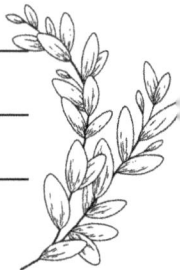

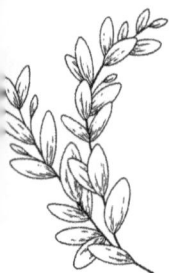

I am grateful for:

Date: _____

_____

_____

_____

_____

_____

_____

_____

Date: _____

_____

_____

_____

_____

_____

_____

_____

I am grateful for:

Date: _____

_____

_____

_____

_____

_____

_____

_____

_____

Date: _____

_____

_____

_____

_____

_____

_____

_____

_____

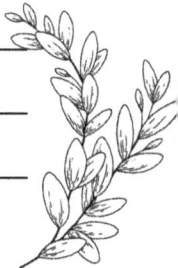

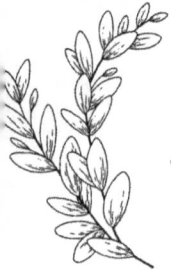

I am grateful for:

Date: _____

_____

_____

_____

_____

_____

_____

_____

Date: _____

_____

_____

_____

_____

_____

_____

_____

Envisioning

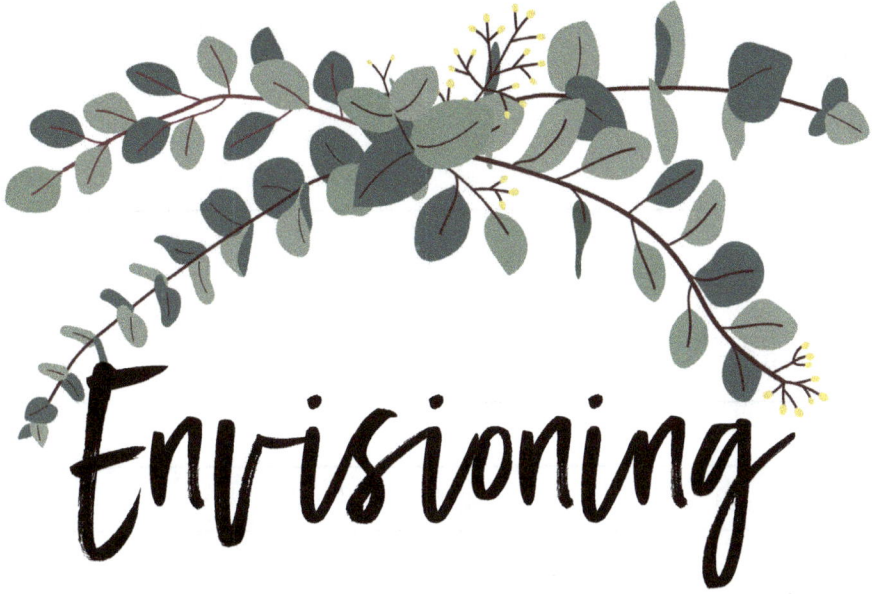

*When I think about my ideal
health, how would I go about
taking one small, realistic
step toward it?*

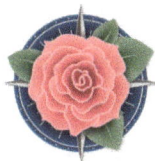

Date: _____

_____

_____

_____

_____

_____

_____

_____

_____

Date: _____

_____

_____

_____

_____

_____

_____

_____

_____

_____

Date: _____

_____

_____

_____

_____

_____

_____

_____

_____

Date: _____

_____

_____

_____

_____

_____

_____

_____

_____

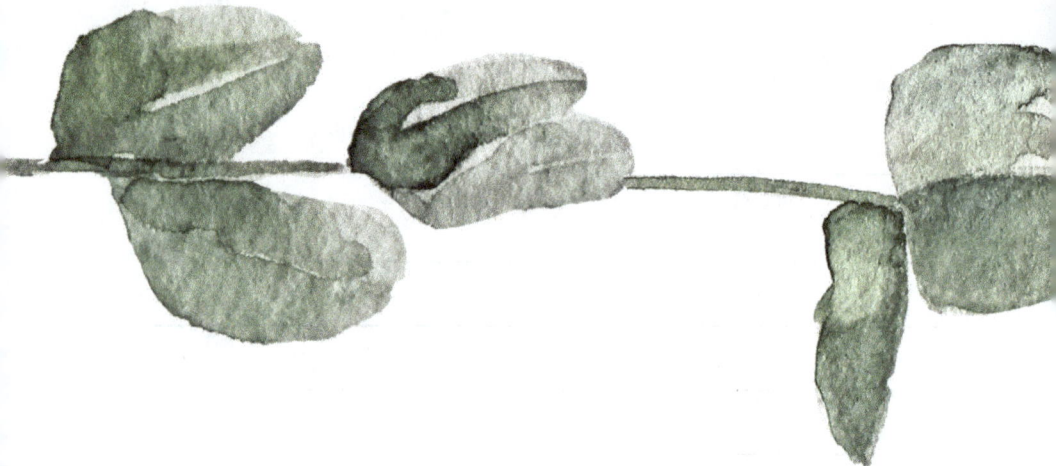

Things happen when we're intentional, specific, and realistic about them.

You can make it an actionable, measurable, and timely goal if it suits you.

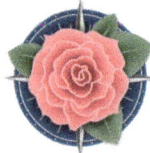

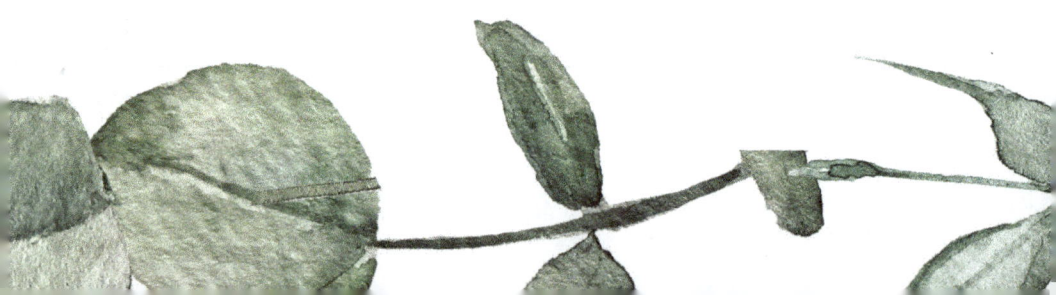

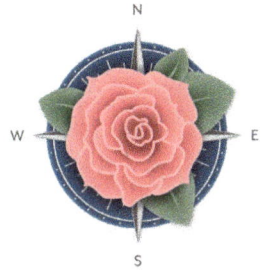

SMART goals have been proved useful toward the success of personal goals.
SMART goals should be:

SPECIFIC. Your goal should be clear and concise. If your goal is not specific, it's hard to see when it begins and when it is complete.

MEASUREABLE. A goal should be measurable so that progress can be tracked. Tracking goals can be inspiring.

ACTION-ORIENTED. A goal should include action. That action should be in your direct control.

REALISTIC. It is best to work with small lifestyle changes that are easy to complete. Focus on small steps at a time.

TIMELY. There should be a timetable for completing the specific, measurable, and realistic actions.

Example: I will walk for 30 minutes/1.5 miles, 5 days a week, outside or on my treadmill.

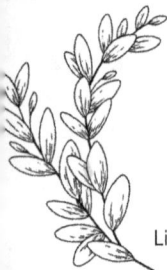

I will be intentional about supporting my mind and body this week by:

List one thing. Try to be as specific and as realistic as possible. Make it a SMART goal.

Week One:

Date: _____

Write goal here.

_____

_____

How did I do?

Write reflection here.

_____

_____

_____

Week Two:

Date: _____

Write goal here.

_____

_____

How did I do?

Write reflection here.

_____

_____

_____

I will be intentional about supporting my mind and body this week by:

List one thing. Try to be as specific and as realistic as possible. Make it a SMART goal.

Week Three:

Date: _____

Write goal here.

_____

_____

How did I do?

Write reflection here.

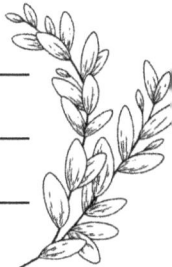

_____

_____

_____

Week Four:

Date: _____

Write goal here.

_____

_____

How did I do?

Write reflection here.

_____

_____

_____

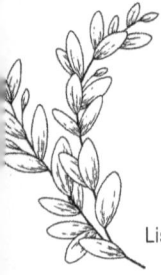

I will be intentional about supporting my mind and body this week by:

List one thing. Try to be as specific and as realistic as possible. Make it a SMART goal.

Week Five:

Date: _____

Write goal here.

_____

_____

How did I do?

Write reflection here.

_____

_____

_____

Week Six:

Date: _____

Write goal here.

_____

_____

How did I do?

Write reflection here.

_____

_____

_____

I will be intentional about supporting
my mind and body this week by:

List one thing. Try to be as specific and as realistic as possible. Make it a SMART goal.

Week Seven:

Date: _____

Write goal here.

_____

_____

How did I do?

Write reflection here.

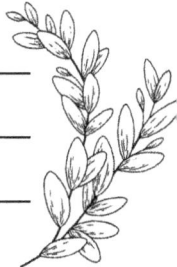

_____

_____

_____

Week Eight:

Date: _____

Write goal here.

_____

_____

How did I do?

Write reflection here.

_____

_____

_____

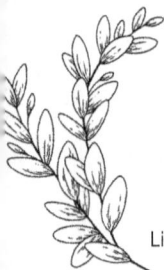

I will be intentional about supporting
my mind and body this week by:

List one thing. Try to be as specific and as realistic as possible. Make it a SMART goal.

Week Nine:

Date: _____

Write goal here.

_____

_____

How did I do?

Write reflection here.

_____

_____

_____

Week Ten:

Date: _____

Write goal here.

_____

_____

How did I do?

Write reflection here.

_____

_____

_____

I will be intentional about supporting my mind and body this week by:

List one thing. Try to be as specific and as realistic as possible. Make it a SMART goal.

Week Eleven:

Date: _____

Write goal here.

_____

_____

How did I do?

Write reflection here.

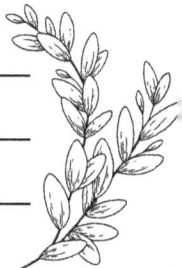

_____

_____

_____

Week Twelve:

Date: _____

Write goal here.

_____

_____

How did I do?

Write reflection here.

_____

_____

_____

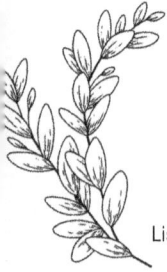

I will be intentional about supporting my mind and body this week by:

List one thing. Try to be as specific and as realistic as possible. Make it a SMART goal.

Week Thirteen:

Date: _____

Write goal here.

_____

_____

How did I do?

Write reflection here.

_____

_____

_____

Week Fourteen:

Date: _____

Write goal here.

_____

_____

How did I do?

Write reflection here.

_____

_____

_____

I will be intentional about supporting
my mind and body this week by:

List one thing. Try to be as specific and as realistic as possible. Make it a SMART goal.

Week Fifteen:

Date: _____

Write goal here.

_____

_____

How did I do?

Write reflection here.

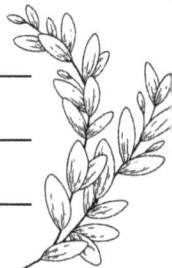

_____

_____

_____

Week Sixteen:

Date: _____

Write goal here.

_____

_____

How did I do?

Write reflection here.

_____

_____

_____

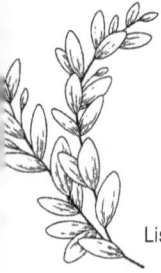

I will be intentional about supporting my mind and body this week by:

List one thing. Try to be as specific and as realistic as possible. Make it a SMART goal.

Week Seventeen:

Date: _____

Write goal here.

_____

_____

How did I do?

Write reflection here.

_____

_____

_____

Week Eighteen:

Date: _____

Write goal here.

_____

_____

How did I do?

Write reflection here.

_____

_____

_____

I will be intentional about supporting
my mind and body this week by:

List one thing. Try to be as specific and as realistic as possible. Make it a SMART goal.

Week Nineteen:

Date: _____

Write goal here.

_____

_____

How did I do?

Write reflection here.

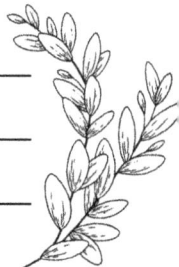

_____

_____

_____

Week Twenty:

Date: _____

Write goal here.

_____

_____

How did I do?

Write reflection here.

_____

_____

_____

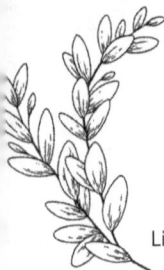

I will be intentional about supporting
my mind and body this week by:

List one thing. Try to be as specific and as realistic as possible. Make it a SMART goal.

Week Twenty-one:

Date: _____

Write goal here.

_____

_____

How did I do?

Write reflection here.

_____

_____

_____

Week Twenty-two:

Date: _____

Write goal here.

_____

_____

How did I do?

Write reflection here.

_____

_____

_____

I will be intentional about supporting my mind and body this week by:

List one thing. Try to be as specific and as realistic as possible. Make it a SMART goal.

Week Twenty-three:

Date: _____

Write goal here.

_____

_____

How did I do?

Write reflection here.

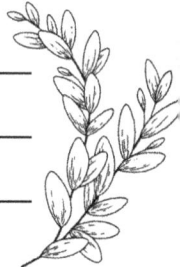

_____

_____

_____

Week Twenty-four:

Date: _____

Write goal here.

_____

_____

How did I do?

Write reflection here.

_____

_____

_____

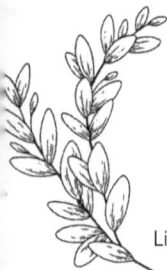

I will be intentional about supporting my mind and body this week by:

List one thing. Try to be as specific and as realistic as possible. Make it a SMART goal.

Week Twenty-five:

Date: _____

Write goal here.

_____

_____

How did I do?

Write reflection here.

_____

_____

_____

Week Twenty-six:

Date: _____

Write goal here.

_____

_____

How did I do?

Write reflection here.

_____

_____

_____

I will be intentional about supporting
my mind and body this week by:

List one thing. Try to be as specific and as realistic as possible. Make it a SMART goal.

Week Twenty-seven:

Date: _____

Write goal here.

_____

_____

How did I do?

Write reflection here.

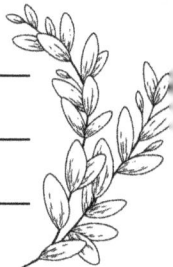

_____

_____

_____

Week Twenty-eight:

Date: _____

Write goal here.

_____

_____

How did I do?

Write reflection here.

_____

_____

_____

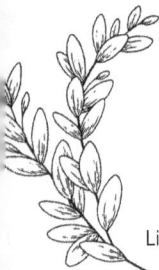

I will be intentional about supporting my mind and body this week by:

List one thing. Try to be as specific and as realistic as possible. Make it a SMART goal.

Week Twenty-nine:

Date: _____

Write goal here.

_____

_____

How did I do?

Write reflection here.

_____

_____

_____

Week Thirty:

Date: _____

Write goal here.

_____

_____

How did I do?

Write reflection here.

_____

_____

_____

I will be intentional about supporting
my mind and body this week by:

List one thing. Try to be as specific and as realistic as possible. Make it a SMART goal.

Week Thirty-one:

Date: _____

Write goal here.

_____

_____

How did I do?

Write reflection here.

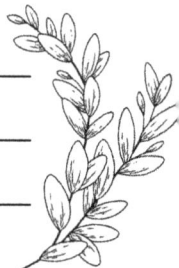

_____

_____

_____

Week Thirty-two:

Date: _____

Write goal here.

_____

_____

How did I do?

Write reflection here.

_____

_____

_____

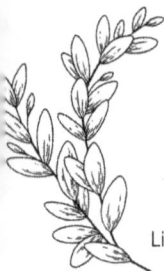

I will be intentional about supporting my mind and body this week by:

List one thing. Try to be as specific and as realistic as possible. Make it a SMART goal.

Week Thirty-three:

Date: _____

Write goal here.

_____

_____

How did I do?

Write reflection here.

_____

_____

_____

Week Thirty-four:

Date: _____

Write goal here.

_____

_____

How did I do?

Write reflection here.

_____

_____

_____

I will be intentional about supporting my mind and body this week by:

List one thing. Try to be as specific and as realistic as possible. Make it a SMART goal.

Week Thirty-five:

Date: _____

Write goal here.

_____

_____

How did I do?

Write reflection here.

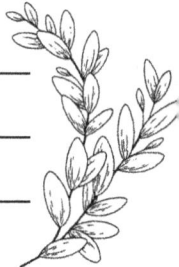

_____

_____

_____

Week Thirty-six:

Date: _____

Write goal here.

_____

_____

How did I do?

Write reflection here.

_____

_____

_____

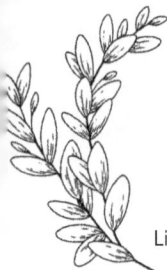

I will be intentional about supporting
my mind and body this week by:

List one thing. Try to be as specific and as realistic as possible. Make it a SMART goal.

Week Thirty-seven:

Date: _____

Write goal here.

_____

_____

How did I do?

Write reflection here.

_____

_____

_____

Week Thirty-eight:

Date: _____

Write goal here.

_____

_____

How did I do?

Write reflection here.

_____

_____

_____

I will be intentional about supporting my mind and body this week by:

List one thing. Try to be as specific and as realistic as possible. Make it a SMART goal.

Week Thirty-nine:

Date: _____

Write goal here.

_____

_____

How did I do?

Write reflection here.

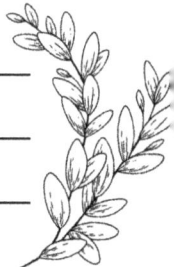

_____

_____

_____

Week Forty:

Date: _____

Write goal here.

_____

_____

How did I do?

Write reflection here.

_____

_____

_____

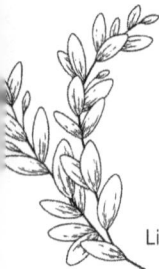

I will be intentional about supporting my mind and body this week by:

List one thing. Try to be as specific and as realistic as possible. Make it a SMART goal.

Week Forty-one:

Date: _____

Write goal here.

_____

_____

How did I do?

Write reflection here.

_____

_____

_____

Week Forty-two:

Date: _____

Write goal here.

_____

_____

How did I do?

Write reflection here.

_____

_____

_____

I will be intentional about supporting my mind and body this week by:

List one thing. Try to be as specific and as realistic as possible. Make it a SMART goal.

Week Forty-three:

Date: _____

Write goal here.

_____

_____

How did I do?

Write reflection here.

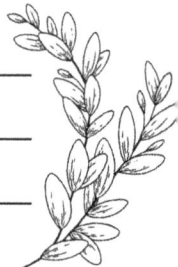

_____

_____

_____

Week Forty-four:

Date: _____

Write goal here.

_____

_____

How did I do?

Write reflection here.

_____

_____

_____

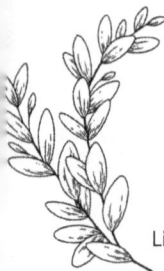

I will be intentional about supporting my mind and body this week by:

List one thing. Try to be as specific and as realistic as possible. Make it a SMART goal.

Week Forty-five:

Date: _____

Write goal here.

_____

_____

How did I do?

Write reflection here.

_____

_____

_____

Week Forty-six:

Date: _____

Write goal here.

_____

_____

How did I do?

Write reflection here.

_____

_____

_____

I will be intentional about supporting my mind and body this week by:

List one thing. Try to be as specific and as realistic as possible. Make it a SMART goal.

Week Forty-seven:

Date: _____

Write goal here.

_____

_____

How did I do?

Write reflection here.

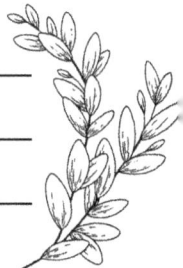

_____

_____

_____

Week Forty-eight:

Date: _____

Write goal here.

_____

_____

How did I do?

Write reflection here.

_____

_____

_____

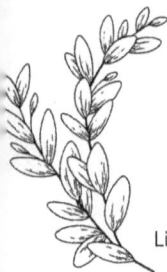

I will be intentional about supporting
my mind and body this week by:

List one thing. Try to be as specific and as realistic as possible. Make it a SMART goal.

Week Forty-nine:

Date: _____

Write goal here.

_____

_____

How did I do?

Write reflection here.

_____

_____

_____

Week Fifty:

Date: _____

Write goal here.

_____

_____

How did I do?

Write reflection here.

_____

_____

_____

I will be intentional about supporting
my mind and body this week by:

List one thing. Try to be as specific and as realistic as possible. Make it a SMART goal.

Week Fifty-one:

Date: _____

Write goal here.

_____

_____

How did I do?

Write reflection here.

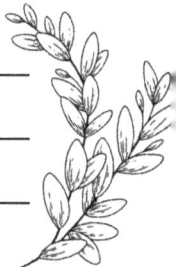

_____

_____

_____

Week Fifty-two:

Date: _____

Write goal here.

_____

_____

How did I do?

Write reflection here.

_____

_____

_____

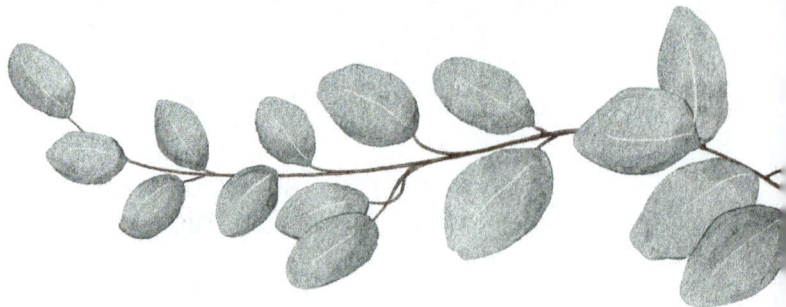

Accomplishments

Use the following pages
to log any accomplishments,
small or big wins.

Celebrate them all.

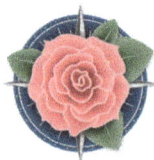

Date: _____

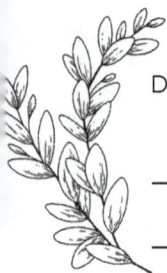

Date: _____

_____

_____

_____

_____

_____

_____

_____

_____

_____

_____

_____

_____

_____

_____

_____

_____

_____

_____

_____

_____

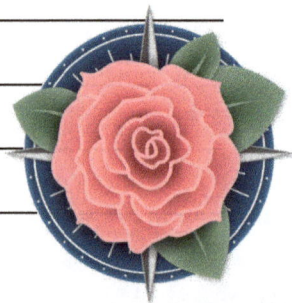

Date: _____

Date: _____

Date: _____

Date: _____

Date: _____

_____

_____

_____

_____

_____

_____

_____

_____

_____

_____

_____

_____

_____

_____

_____

_____

_____

_____

_____

_____

Date: _____

Date: _____

Date: _____

Date: _____

_____

_____

_____

_____

_____

_____

_____

_____

_____

_____

_____

_____

_____

_____

_____

_____

_____

_____

_____

_____

_____

_____

_____

Date: _____

Date: _____

_____

_____

_____

_____

_____

_____

_____

_____

_____

_____

_____

_____

_____

_____

_____

_____

_____

_____

_____

_____

_____

_____

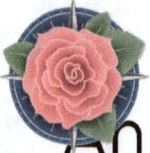

An Excercise about joy

Now, compare the lists. What stands out to me?
Is there anything I can do to adjust my day-to-day life?

Self-Care Bingo

May this inspire some self-care practices in your world.
Create a BINGO line and keep going.

B	I	N	G	O
MAKE A GRATITUDE LIST	COMPLIMENT SOMEONE	READ A POSITIVE AFFIRMATION	WORKOUT	DECLUTTER ONE SPACE
TRY SOMETHING NEW	SPEAK TO SOMEONE WHO NOURISHES YOUR SOUL	HYDRATE WITH PLENTY OF WATER	GET A FULL NIGHT'S REST	HUG A PET OR A LOVED ONE OR TELL SOMEONE HOW MUCH YOU CARE ABOUT THEM
CREATE SOMETHING	ESCAPE INTO A GOOD BOOK FOR FUN		PRACTICE SELF-COMPASSION	SPEND TIME OUTSIDE
GO FOR A WALK	TAKE A SOCIAL MEDIA BREAK	WATCH A MOVIE	TAKE A NAP	COMPLETE A MEDITATION PRACTICE
PREPARE A NUTRITIOUS MEAL	STRETCH FOR 10 MINUTES	JOURNAL ABOUT ANYTHING	DO A MINDFUL PRACTICE	GIVE YOURSELF A COMPLIMENT

Journaling prompts for each dimension of health

Choose any prompt that speaks to you and write about it on any blank pages throughout the journal.

Nutrition

What healthy foods do I eat that make my body feel good?

Movement

What activities do I engage in that support my cardiovascular health, my strength, and my flexibility?

Rest

What does a day of rest look like? How can I create that for myself?

Mental/Emotional

Am I holding on to something I need to let go of?

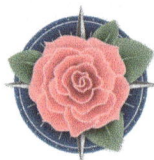

Journaling prompts for each dimension of health

Social Life & Relationships

What are the relationships in my life that fill me up vs. drain me? How can I make more time for the ones that fill me up?

Spirituality

What is one spiritual practice that serves me? Am I doing it enough? If not, how can I make time for more?

Physical Environment

What is one space in my home/office/etc. that can use some sprucing up? How can I make it a healthier environment for myself?

Personal & Professional Development

If money and time were no object, what would I love to do that would bring me a profound sense of satisfaction, joy, and purpose?

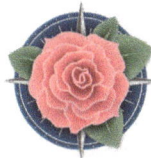

Other journaling prompts I may like

- How can I create more self-confidence for myself?

- What is my main focus this week?

- What do I need to do to finish this week off strong?

- What activity did I most enjoy doing when I was younger? Can I incorporate it into my life now?

- What's been my best experience with my health goals this week?

- How am I taking care of me today?

- When was the last time I did something creative?

- What am I most proud of this week?

- Who in my life are the most supportive people to be around?

- What is currently bringing me joy?

- What am I feeding my mind? Does it align with how I want to feel?

- How can I bring my best to others today?

- What part of my job is the most fun?

- Who are the positive people in my life?

- What am I most grateful for today?

- What are beliefs I have about my health that limit me? How can I overcome this?

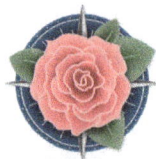

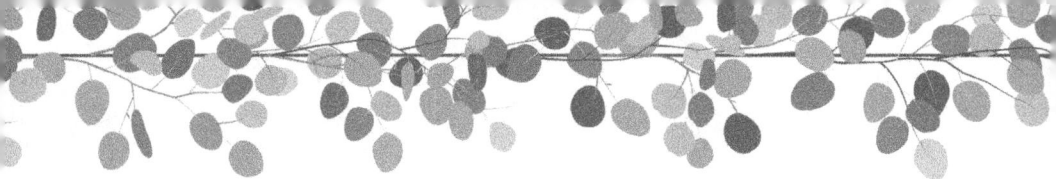

- What do I want my health for?

- What are my top priorities right now?

- What makes me feel optimistic about my future?

- What keeps me grounded?

- What is one thing that made me smile today?

- What will I do this week for self-care?

- What do I do to relax?

- What is one book that has supported my well-being?

- How do I enjoy spending time on my own?

- Who are the people who encourage me and share in my happy news?

- Who are positive influences in my life?

- What do I most need today?

- What am I most proud of this week?

- What do I need to let go of to support my health?

- What negative habits am I ready to break?

- What current habits are most serving me?

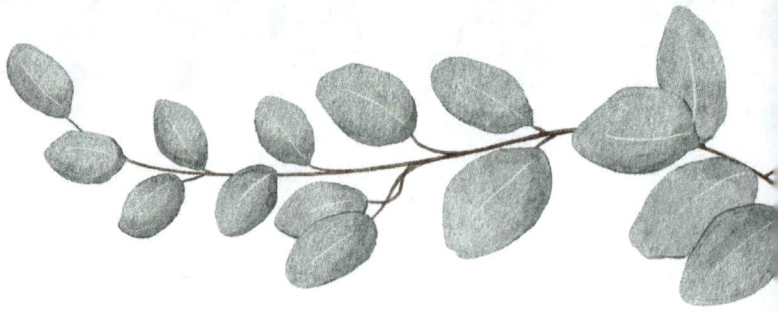

Freestyle
journaling

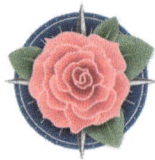

Date: _____

Date: _____

_____

_____

_____

_____

_____

_____

_____

_____

_____

_____

_____

_____

_____

_____

_____

_____

_____

_____

_____

_____

Date: _____

_____

_____

_____

_____

_____

_____

_____

_____

_____

_____

_____

_____

_____

_____

_____

_____

_____

_____

_____

_____

_____

_____

Date: _____

Date: _____

_____

_____

_____

_____

_____

_____

_____

_____

_____

_____

_____

_____

_____

_____

_____

_____

_____

_____

_____

_____

_____

_____

_____

Date: _____

_____

_____

_____

_____

_____

_____

_____

_____

_____

_____

_____

_____

_____

_____

_____

_____

_____

_____

_____

Date: _____

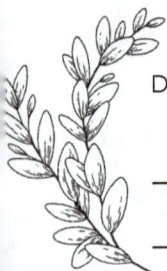

Date: _____

_____

_____

_____

_____

_____

_____

_____

_____

_____

_____

_____

_____

_____

_____

_____

_____

_____

_____

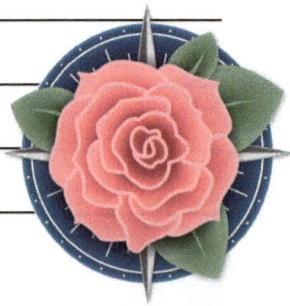

Date: _____

Date: _____

Date: _____

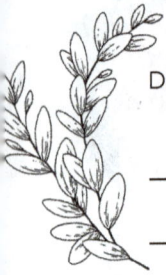

Date: _____

_____

_____

_____

_____

_____

_____

_____

_____

_____

_____

_____

_____

_____

_____

_____

_____

_____

_____

_____

_____

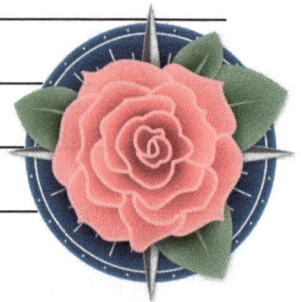

Date: _____

_____

_____

_____

_____

_____

_____

_____

_____

_____

_____

_____

_____

_____

_____

_____

_____

_____

_____

_____

_____

_____

_____

_____

_____

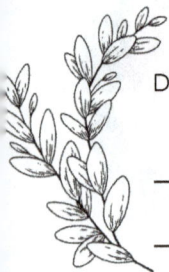

Date: _____

_____

_____

_____

_____

_____

_____

_____

_____

_____

_____

_____

_____

_____

_____

_____

_____

_____

_____

_____

_____

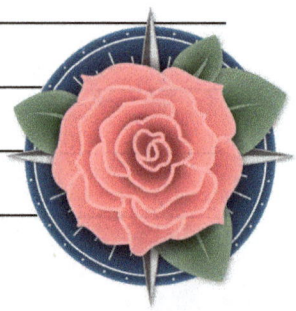

Date: _____

_____

_____

_____

_____

_____

_____

_____

_____

_____

_____

_____

_____

_____

_____

_____

_____

_____

_____

_____

_____

_____

_____

_____

Date: _____

Date: _____

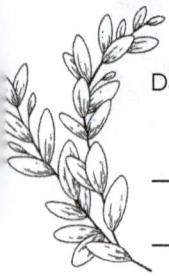

Date: _____

_____

_____

_____

_____

_____

_____

_____

_____

_____

_____

_____

_____

_____

_____

_____

_____

_____

_____

_____

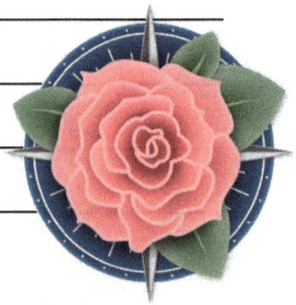

Date: _____

_____

_____

_____

_____

_____

_____

_____

_____

_____

_____

_____

_____

_____

_____

_____

_____

_____

_____

_____

_____

_____

_____

Date: _____

Date: _____

_____

_____

_____

_____

_____

_____

_____

_____

_____

_____

_____

_____

_____

_____

_____

_____

_____

_____

_____

_____

_____

_____

_____

Date: _____

Date: _____

_____

_____

_____

_____

_____

_____

_____

_____

_____

_____

_____

_____

_____

_____

_____

_____

_____

_____

_____

_____

_____

_____

_____

Date: _____

Date: _____

_____

_____

_____

_____

_____

_____

_____

_____

_____

_____

_____

_____

_____

_____

_____

_____

_____

_____

_____

_____

_____

_____

Date: _____

_____

_____

_____

_____

_____

_____

_____

_____

_____

_____

_____

_____

_____

_____

_____

_____

_____

_____

Date: _____

_____

_____

_____

_____

_____

_____

_____

_____

_____

_____

_____

_____

_____

_____

_____

_____

_____

_____

_____

_____

_____

_____

_____

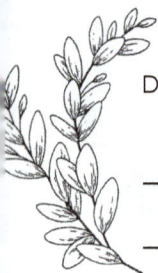

Date: _____

_____

_____

_____

_____

_____

_____

_____

_____

_____

_____

_____

_____

_____

_____

_____

_____

_____

_____

_____

_____

_____

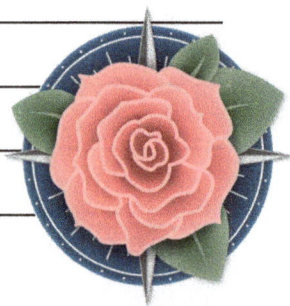

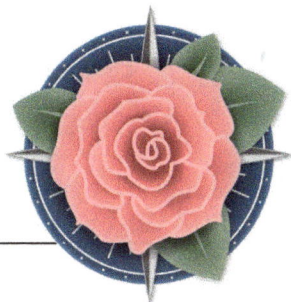

Date: _____

_____

_____

_____

_____

_____

_____

_____

_____

_____

_____

_____

_____

_____

_____

_____

_____

_____

_____

_____

_____

_____

_____

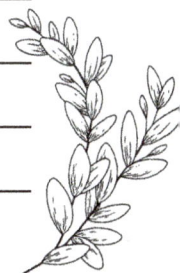

Date: _____

Date: _____

Date: _____

Date: _____

_____

_____

_____

_____

_____

_____

_____

_____

_____

_____

_____

_____

_____

_____

_____

_____

_____

_____

_____

_____

_____

_____

_____

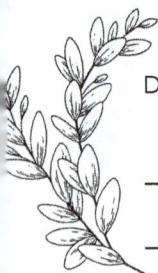

Date: _____

_____

_____

_____

_____

_____

_____

_____

_____

_____

_____

_____

_____

_____

_____

_____

_____

_____

_____

_____

_____

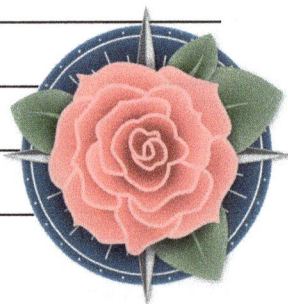

Date: _____

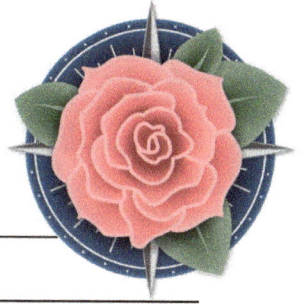

_____

_____

_____

_____

_____

_____

_____

_____

_____

_____

_____

_____

_____

_____

_____

_____

_____

_____

_____

_____

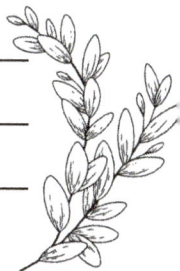

Date: _____

Date: _____

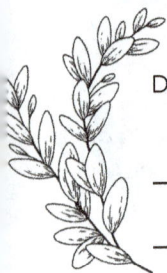

Date: _____

_____

_____

_____

_____

_____

_____

_____

_____

_____

_____

_____

_____

_____

_____

_____

_____

_____

_____

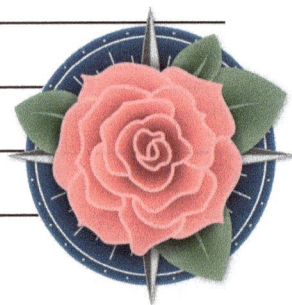

Date: _____

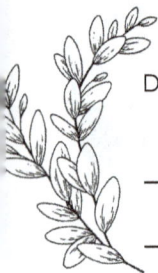

Date: _____

_____

_____

_____

_____

_____

_____

_____

_____

_____

_____

_____

_____

_____

_____

_____

_____

_____

_____

_____

_____

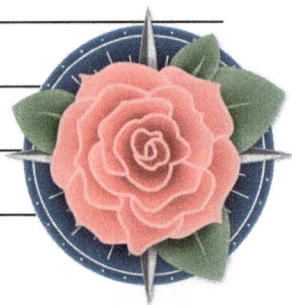

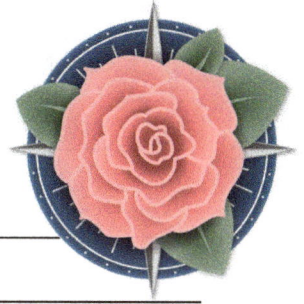

Date: _____

_____
_____
_____
_____
_____
_____
_____
_____
_____
_____
_____
_____
_____
_____
_____
_____
_____
_____
_____
_____
_____
_____

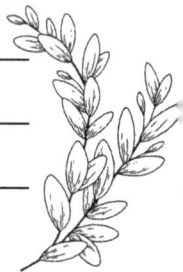

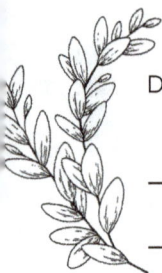

Date: _____

_____

_____

_____

_____

_____

_____

_____

_____

_____

_____

_____

_____

_____

_____

_____

_____

_____

_____

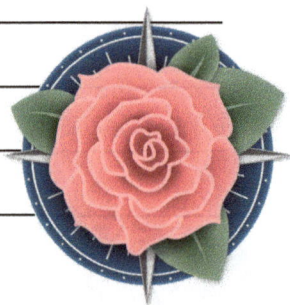

Date: _____

_____

_____

_____

_____

_____

_____

_____

_____

_____

_____

_____

_____

_____

_____

_____

_____

_____

_____

_____

_____

_____

_____

Date: _____

_____

_____

_____

_____

_____

_____

_____

_____

_____

_____

_____

_____

_____

_____

_____

_____

_____

_____

_____

_____

Date: _____

_____

_____

_____

_____

_____

_____

_____

_____

_____

_____

_____

_____

_____

_____

_____

_____

_____

_____

_____

_____

_____

_____

_____

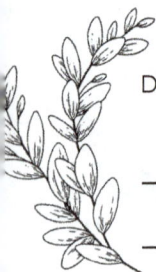

Date: _____

_____

_____

_____

_____

_____

_____

_____

_____

_____

_____

_____

_____

_____

_____

_____

_____

_____

_____

_____

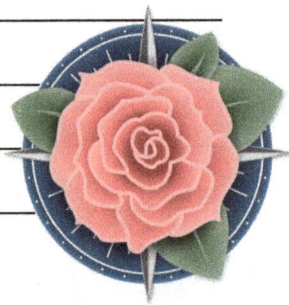

Date: _____

_____

_____

_____

_____

_____

_____

_____

_____

_____

_____

_____

_____

_____

_____

_____

_____

_____

_____

_____

_____

Date: _____

Date: _____

_____

_____

_____

_____

_____

_____

_____

_____

_____

_____

_____

_____

_____

_____

_____

_____

_____

_____

_____

_____

_____

About the Author

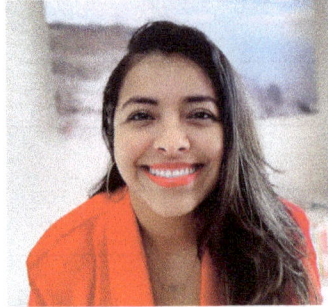

Rosy Crumpton, NBC-HWC

*R*osy is a firm believer that we have the power to achieve our best health. Through a supportive partnership, she helps people set and achieve goals they most want in life to help lead a happy, healthy, and more balanced life.

With a bachelor's degree in psychology and professional experience in behavioral healthcare since 2005, Rosy is knowledgeable on what it takes to create behavioral change. She was trained at Duke Health and Well-Being, previously known as Duke Integrative Medicine, where she received her Integrative Health Coaching course and Certification, on a whole person care health approach. She is a National Board Certified Health & Wellness Coach, a robust certification which represents the profession's highest standard.

Rosy feels passionate about helping people who could benefit from a little structure and guidance on envisioning and carrying out their personal and professional wellness goals. She feels strongly about autonomy of choice by honoring each individual for their strengths, choices, past experiences, and how they want to make change.

She is a professional writer and speaker who loves to read, cook, and advocate for her community. She's the founder and CEO of Sophrosyne Wellness. She lives in Matthews, North Carolina where she spends time with her husband Brandon and their cat baby Arya.

Connect with Rosy.
www.rosycrumpton.com
www.sophrosynewellness.com

www.ingramcontent.com/pod-product-compliance
Lightning Source LLC
Chambersburg PA
CBHW072125090426
42739CB00012B/3064